The Wuhan Coronavirus

Survival Manual and Concise Guide to COVID-19 (Symptoms, Outbreak, and Prevention in 2020)

Robert Miller

Table of Contents

Introduction

The coronavirus outbreak has been a topic of frequent contention since it began in December of 2019. The virus, also referred to as the novel coronavirus and COVID-19, is not the first coronavirus we have seen; the virus that caused severe acute respiratory syndrome (SARS) was also a type of coronavirus, as was Middle East respiratory syndrome (MERS). Though it is not the first of its kind, the current strain of coronavirus has led to a great deal of anxiety, panic, and often misrepresentation as a result. Some sources may downplay how likely it is for anyone to catch the coronavirus, which could lead to people failing to seek medical treatment, while other sources may dramatize the virus' effects in an attempt to draw attention, creating pandemonium and oftentimes resulting in harmful stereotypes that do nothing to keep people safe.

If we want to take the proper precautions to keep ourselves healthy during the coronavirus outbreak and know what to do should we or someone we know become infected, we must know all we can about the virus. This means cutting through the many myths surrounding the coronavirus and having a good idea of the truth of the matter. It is only through an honest representation of the threat that we can understand what we are facing and how we can go about protecting ourselves from it. Knowledge is incredibly valuable during an outbreak, and the more we understand, the less likely we are to believe the obfuscation of the facts that occurs in a great deal of the current coronavirus coverage.

In order to fully understand the coronavirus, we must first have an understanding of viruses and how they operate within the body.

An Introduction to Virology

Virology is the study of exactly what viruses are and what effects they have on us, specifically at the individual cell level. Viruses are microscopic particles, meaning they cannot be seen by the human eye. Despite this, they can be one of the most dangerous things we encounter on a day to day basis. A virus is made up of two main components. The first is the virus' genetic code or genome, which can be made of either ribonucleic acid (RNA) or deoxyribonucleic acid (DNA). This is what infects the cell and provides the new material for it to replicate instead of the normal cell DNA. The other part is the protein capsid, which forms a protective outer layer for the virus. The capsid layer allows viruses to survive in our bodies for long enough to interact with one of our cells.

Viruses enter our system and target vulnerable cells, which they then take over and convert to virus replication factories. They can turn a perfectly healthy cell into one that needs to be destroyed by your immune system for your body to return to its normal functions and fight off an illness. Once a virus is in the body, how does it complete this process?

First, the virus injects its genome into a host cell. Infected cells are usually specific to the type of virus; for example, a virus known for producing upper respiratory symptoms like wheezing and shortness of breath may only target cells in the respiratory system, like those in your lungs. It may be unable to affect cells in, say, your stomach lining. However, some viruses have a wider spread and are not as specialized, meaning they can infect most cells of the body and sometimes may be able to infect multiple species. One the genome has been injected into the cell, the new DNA or RNA overrides whatever previous activity the cell was doing in the body. At this point, the host cell begins replicating the virus genome instead of its own genome, which causes it to make more and more viruses. At a certain point, the host cell will burst, sending these newly formed viruses out into the rest of the body to repeat the process on a larger scale.

Our bodies are not completely defenseless against this takeover. Our immune system works to fight off many harmful foreign agents, including bacteria and viruses. Your immune system contains B cells and T cells, each of which plays a role in providing protection. Your B cells patrol your body and signal when something potentially harmful is discovered, and then attempt to neutralize it. This is accomplished through antibodies, which are produced in response to a specific harmful agent identified by your B cells. The recognition process is aided if your body has come into contact with the specific virus before, as antibodies for the virus and the B cells that make them will already be circulating through your system. This is why vaccines help us to fight against viruses, as they expose our B cells to a very limited amount of a virus without risk of infection. Once recognized, antibodies bind to these harmful foreign components, called antigens, and suppress their ability to affect your health. They also provide a signal that is recognized by T cells, which then come to destroy the antigen.

The destruction of an infected cell is known as cell lysing, where the cell pops and it no longer continues replication processes. While this is useful to your body for dealing with cells containing viruses, it is also used on a regular basis for cells that are too old or that have deviated from their standard functions in some other way. It may sound like you will be dealing with a cell deficit, but your body contains around 30 trillion cells, so under typical circumstances it is unlikely for you to be in any danger of running out of a given type of cell. Still, viruses can become an issue in your body due to their exponential replication, which allows them to affect a large number of your cells if they are not stopped by your immune system.

Despite the danger they pose to us, it is important to keep in mind that viruses are not operating this way on purpose. In fact, most scientists agree that viruses aren't even technically alive. They do not act maliciously, nor do they actively 'choose' who to infect and who not to infect. The only thing driving a virus is its instinct to survive and replicate, which means that the only way to prevent a virus from infecting as many cells as it can is to lyse the infected cells, and therefore destroy the virus. Failure to do so can lead to illness, the transfer of the virus from one person to many others, and eventually an outbreak if the virus is not managed in time.

Outbreak Terminology

You may have heard terms like outbreak, epidemic, and pandemic in reference to the coronavirus, but what do these terms actually mean? Is there a big difference between a virus that is considered a pandemic and one that is considered an epidemic? Many sources use these terms interchangeably with little concern for their true meanings. Still, it is a good idea to know the differences so you can know how the current coronavirus outbreak should be classified at this point in time.

An outbreak is the least specific identifier of a larger than normal number of cases of a disease. They may be caused by infections or by mass exposure to a certain harmful chemical. There is no specified number or rate for something to be considered an outbreak, so it can be used fairly generally. An outbreak may be as few as a few hundred cases concentrated in a small area, or it may be as many as thousands across the globe. It simply refers to more than usual. This means that something like the influenza virus, that infects tens of thousands of people each year, may not be considered an outbreak because this is the expected number of cases. The flu would only be classified as an outbreak if there were an excess of cases overall, or if there were many more cases than usual in a given area. At this point, it is safe to call the coronavirus an outbreak, as the thousands of cases currently on record surpass the 'normal' number, which would be few to none.

An epidemic involves a very rapid spread of a certain disease. It usually refers to a time period of about two weeks; infection outbreaks that do not make it for this long are generally not elevated to the status of an epidemic. Epidemics also refer to specific geographic areas. Though the coronavirus may not currently be an epidemic in the United States, as there have not yet been enough cases to classify it as such, it could be said to be an epidemic in places like China and Italy which have a much higher density of cases.

Many people confuse 'epidemic' with the similar sounding term 'endemic,' but while they can both refer to viral infections, these terms are not to be used interchangeably. If a disease is endemic, it is typical to a certain area or group of people, and it is generally not an easily transmittable global concern like the coronavirus. Endemic can be used to describe things other than viruses as well. For example, the kangaroo is a species that is endemic to Australia. This does not mean that it cannot exist elsewhere should certain circumstances occur, such as kangaroos at the zoo, but you are much more likely to see a kangaroo in Australia than you are to see one in Florida. Similarly, diseases that are endemic are much more common in one area than another.

The term pandemic refers to a disease that spreads across a wide region. This usually has a more global connotation, such as a disease that exists across many different countries and has spread to multiple continents. Though not caused by viral origins, the black plague is considered to have been a pandemic, as is the viral spanish influenza that occurred in 1918. For a great deal of its existence, the coronavirus was not considered to be a pandemic, though its fairly large spread and its tendency to be transmitted across borders had many wondering if it would become one in the near future. Its designation changed very recently, on March 11, to pandemic status as the virus found more footholds in countries around the globe.

Now that you understand the terminology surrounding viruses, we can move on to getting a better idea of the coronavirus specifically and what the current pandemic means for those affected.

Chapter 1: Understanding the Coronavirus

You likely have many unanswered questions about the coronavirus and what it means for your health. It can be hard to know how worried you should be about a potential infection and, should you contract the virus, how likely you are to survive. By breaking down the virus and gaining a better understanding of it, we can get a better idea of what sort of danger it poses and what we should be doing to keep our chances of contracting the virus as low as possible. With the right information, keeping yourself safe and healthy becomes much more likely, even if you are very close to an area experiencing an outbreak. Of course, there is little to no way to guarantee you do not become sick provided you are not willing or able to completely isolate yourself, but even taking a few small steps can help to improve the likelihood of avoiding infection or making a full recovery should you become exposed to the virus.

First, it is necessary to look at what exactly a coronavirus is and how and where it is believed to have started. Next, we will tackle some of the commonly reported symptoms and develop an understanding of the ways the virus travels between people so you can know what to avoid and what is safe. Finally, we will discuss how you can lower your chances of getting sick and what you should do if you believe your illness may be a product of the coronavirus.

What Is a Coronavirus?

A coronavirus is not just one virus but a series of hundreds of similar viruses. A coronavirus is named after the appearance of the virus under a microscope. It is circular with small spikes around the exterior, which protrude to look like the points on a crown. Since the latin word for crown is 'corona,' the crown-shaped virus was dubbed the coronavirus. The majority of coronaviruses simply lead to cold symptoms and do not have any especially communicative or deadly effects. There are a few notable exceptions to this rule, which are the coronaviruses that have become the most well known.

The most infectious and dangerous coronaviruses are either more resilient to our immune systems or they impact more vulnerable parts of our bodies. Different coronaviruses are capable of producing different proteins which might make them better equipped to fight back against our antibodies. This means a very strong immune system is needed to combat these viruses, which in turn means more people with average and weakened immune systems are infected. It also means that even in healthy people, the risk of developing a more severe fever from the heightened immune system response is much higher. Some coronaviruses are more concerning because they impact parts of the bodies that are at a bigger risk of malfunctioning. Less dangerous viruses target cells "higher up in the respiratory tract — places like your nose or throat," while more worrying strains "attach in the lungs and bronchial tubes, causing more serious infections" (Harrison, 2020, para. 18). The current coronavirus seems to be more troublesome than the common cold, which indicates it is likely attaching in areas like the lower respiratory tract, which makes it harder for your body to deal with. It may also be applying additional strain to the immune system. Not much is known about the exact proteins COVID-19 produces or how adept they are at fighting off our immune systems just yet. Further research will likely provide the answers to these questions as time goes on.

Other Coronaviruses

As previously mentioned, COVID-19 is not the first coronavirus outbreak we have experienced. While there are many types of coronaviruses, not all of them can infect humans, and many of the ones that do are not able to severely impact people with average immune systems. However, there are some exceptions. Two notable examples are SARS and MERS, which both had well known outbreaks within the last 20 years.

The SARS outbreak began in February of 2003. The first cases were identified in Asia, and from there spread to many different countries, largely as a result of unknowing travel to infected areas and close contact with people who had the virus. It lasted for about six months, and in that time infected over 8,000 people and led to just under 800 deaths.

MERS first appeared in 2012, but the largest outbreak did not occur until 2015. As the name suggests, it tends to appear in the Middle East, with all cases being connected to the area of the Arabian Peninsula. Though the 2015 outbreak occurred in the Republic of Korea, it was brought to the area by someone who had recently traveled to the Arabian Peninsula. The death rate of MERS is quite a bit higher than SARS, with around three or four cases out of every 10 resulting in deaths (CDC, 2019, para. 1). This is triple or quadruple the average mortality rate for SARS.

Source of the Coronavirus

The current coronavirus strain is zoonotic, which means it began in animals and then spread to humans. This is believed to have occurred in a meat market in Wuhan, where many people came into close contact with animals, both alive and dead, that may have been infected with coronaviruses. There has been some debate as to the exact animal the virus came from. At first pangolins, which are scale-covered anteaters, were suspected to be the source. However, later reports have also suggested animals such as bats and civet cats. The most likely contender is bats, which are known to carry many other strains of coronavirus, some of which are very similar to the one currently infecting humans.

Even though animal sources are believed to have caused the initial infection, the vast majority of succeeding infections have occurred between two humans. There is little reason to be concerned over catching the virus from an animal, especially if you do not live within China; at this point, it is much more likely that you would catch the coronavirus from another person than an animal. Staple protein sources like chicken, beef, and pork have all been deemed safe to eat at this time.

Risk Factors

While no one is immune to the virus, some people are more at risk of catching it than others. The reasons why can be explained in two ways. The first is location based; people who are closer to areas with a higher density of confirmed cases are going to be more likely to contract the virus than those who are more isolated. The second is individual health factors that may put you more at risk for either catching the coronavirus or experiencing more severe symptoms than the typical case. Both of these factors are things to consider when evaluating your personal risk level and deciding on your plan of action.

High Risk Areas

The most high risk areas are those that currently have many cases of coronavirus. This of course includes the epicenter of the virus in China, especially Wuhan and the surrounding area. Currently there is a quarantine on Wuhan, so it is unlikely that the zone poses an active threat to those outside the quarantine, but anyone who was recently in the area may be at risk. Chinese residents may be more likely to contract coronavirus because of their proximity to the virus' origins and the way the virus has continued to spread throughout the country.

The quarantine in Wuhan is just one component of the Chinese government's attempts to contain the virus. Aggressive containment measures in other areas of China have attempted to keep the spread as small as possible as well. With these measures in place, it is likely that the majority of cross country spread of the virus occurred within the early days, before it became an international concern and quarantines were put in place, and further spread is occurring due to those who have traveled to areas of infection and unknowingly brought the virus back with them. Doctors and researchers in China have also begun deploying experimental treatments and new research methods in an effort to develop either a reliable cure or a preventative vaccine sometime in the future.

Despite being the most well-known location of the virus, China is not the only place experts have advised restricted travel for. Italy is experiencing a severe outbreak, with a great deal of its population infected. It is recommended that, when possible, you should avoid traveling to Italy for the duration of the outbreak. Iran, South Korea, and Japan are also suggesting that people limit their traveling. By limiting the number of people entering and leaving the country, fewer people become exposed to the virus, leading to less ability for the virus to spread into countries that are entire plane or boat rides away.

Within the United States, there are fewer cases of the virus but there are still areas that have been hit harder than others. Currently, California has expressed concerns over a steadily growing number of cases, which means west coast residents may be more at risk than the rest of the country at this time. Still, there have been a few reported cases in different states throughout the country, totaling just under 200 at present. Check local news reports for the most current updates on if there have been confirmed cases within your area.

The United States has taken its own measures to protect people from the virus as well. This involves carefully monitoring people who have been on planes and cruise ships and, in some areas, imposing short quarantines on people who have traveled from areas with a high infection density. Funding has also been diverted to support hospitals, research, and other medical facilities working to combat the virus. The government came to an agreement "on an $8.3 billion measure to battle the coronavirus outbreak" (Taylor, 2020, para. 1) in early March. This is a result of the virus' area of effect continuing to grow within the country throughout the last month. With these precautions alongside those being taken by other countries, governments hope to keep those who are still healthy away from possible sources of infection and contain the coronavirus before it can spread past already existing high risk areas.

High Risk Health Factors

Location is not the only factor that matters when it comes to your likelihood of being infected. Even in high infection density areas, not every resident is infected. This is because some peoples' bodies are better equipped to fight off viruses depending on their physical states. Certain factors can make you more susceptible to catching and being hit harder by the coronavirus. One of these factors is age. Very young children tend to pick up illnesses more easily because their immune systems are still learning to fight off many bacteria and viruses that we encounter every day. This puts added strain on their immune systems, which can impede their ability to mount a response against the coronavirus. Conversely, elderly people are at a heightened risk for contracting the disease and may be more likely to experience severe symptoms because our immune systems tend to become weaker after a certain point in our lives. They may be less efficient at making new antibodies or even have trouble replicating existing antibodies. A weakened immune system leaves people less capable of fighting off the coronavirus once encountered. This is true of other viruses like the flu as well, which is why it is often recommended that people over the age of 65 get flu shots at the beginning of the season.

There are other reasons why someone may be immunocompromised. They may have contracted a virus that impacts the efficiency of their immune system such as HIV or AIDS, which leaves them more vulnerable to future infections. People who experienced malnutrition, especially during childhood development, experience higher rates of immunodeficiency as well. Poor sanitary habits can also contribute to a higher likelihood of contracting the virus.

Even those with immune system deficiencies or close proximity to areas of infection are not guaranteed to get infected. While you should certainly practice higher levels of vigilance should you fall into one of these categories, it does not mean you should assume that there is no hope. Having one or more high risk factors does not have to mean that you are fated to get sick, and many people in similar situations either do not get sick at all or make full recoveries. Still, should these criteria apply to you, you should pay attention to your health and take note of any unusual symptoms that may be cause to seek medical treatment.

Coronavirus Symptoms

If you believe you may be in danger of contracting the virus, knowing the symptoms can help you have a more certain idea of whether or not you are ill. Responding quickly to a potential infection is important, and failing to know what typical coronavirus symptoms look like can lead to the virus growing into a less manageable problem.

The typical symptoms are usually respiratory related issues. These can include sneezing, coughing, and more severe wheezing. In some cases, infected patients may experience a shortness of breath or tightness in their chest that impacts their ability to breathe. Fever is another signifier to look out for; some may be mild, with only a few tenths of a degree difference from your typical temperature, while others may be severe. Fever and respiratory issues can lead to fatigue and high levels of exhaustion. If left untreated, they can develop into pneumonia, which poses a real threat to those who have been infected. Symptoms generally occur within two weeks of viral exposure, after which you can be fairly likely you will not be impacted by the disease.

Unfortunately, the symptoms for the coronavirus are not very specific to this specific virus. There is a good amount of crossover with cold viruses and influenza symptoms. One of the key identifiers of coronavirus is conditions like coming into contact with someone else with the infection or traveling to an area with many infected people. For example, if you recently returned from a trip to Italy and begin to experience the above symptoms, you may reasonably believe you have caught the coronavirus; the same is true if someone at your workplace was diagnosed with it. If, however, there have been no confirmed cases yet in your state and you have not done much traveling, the chances for your symptoms to be a product of a severe cold are fairly high. Still, it is best to keep an eye on these symptoms and see if they develop, as you may have unknowingly been exposed to the virus.

Even if you recognize some of the symptoms and you believe you may be at risk of contracting the coronavirus, you may not know when it is appropriate or necessary to see a doctor. Fairly mild symptoms, like a light cough or a runny nose, can be by and large dealt with at home with some over the counter medication for your symptoms. If you are likely to recover on your own, it is better to stay home and not risk being further exposed or spreading the virus to more people. If your symptoms worsen, or if you have an immune system deficiency, you should seek treatment to prevent the worsening symptoms from developing into pneumonia or resulting organ damage.

Methods of Transmission

There is an important reason why, unlike many other diseases, people with mild symptoms they can treat themselves are being encouraged to remain at home rather than leaving the house for a doctor's office or hospital. This is because the coronavirus has a high rate of transmission. It seems to spread very quickly and easily, and just one infected person in a public space could lead to many people catching the coronavirus. Learning about the virus' methods of transmission can help you avoid contracting it from others and, should you catch it yourself, allow you to do your part in limiting others' exposure.

Animal to Human

The rate of transfer between animals and humans is very low. Bats are the animal most likely to transmit COVID-19; luckily, few people rarely come into contact with bats, and those that do are still not especially likely to contract the disease.

The virus may have originated in bats, but bats are not spreading the virus. It is probably not too difficult for the majority of people to limit their contact with potentially infected bats, so if you can restrict the time you spend in close contact with potential animal transmitters, it is best practice to do so.

Human to Human

The main method of coronavirus spread is between people. Initially, many cases were a result of direct contact with people who were sick. Travelers may have brought the disease back with them, which is how a virus with an otherwise restricted radius might cross seas. As more people are infected, the primary method of transmission shifts away from direct contact. When the virus continues to infect those with little to no connection to infected areas, it spreads through community transmission. It is what may make going out in public in a quarantined zone a poor choice, even if the area is nowhere near the original site of infection. Coronavirus cases occur as part of a continuous chain. One traveler may bring back the virus and spread it to two other people, who in turn spread it to more who have no direct contact with the original traveler, and who may not even know the people they happen to get the virus from well. The virus proceeds to spread throughout the community, jumping between people with no relationships to each other that have shared spaces.

The exact method for how the virus moves from one person to another is most frequently though close contact with an infected person. When someone with the virus coughs or sneezes, small droplets from their respiratory system may enter another person's system through the eyes, nose, and mouth. Alternatively, they may land on a surface that is later touched by others without being disinfected. This can lead to an infection if the person then touches their face or does not wash their hands before a meal. It is important to follow proper health and safety precautions to keep yourself free of infection.

Preventing Infection

We have already discussed that certain locations and health conditions can increase your chances of catching the virus. While you cannot directly control your age or your immune system strength, you can still take steps to keep yourself safe if you are immunocompromised. If possible, remove yourself from areas that are experiencing outbreaks. This is not always an option, but if you can stay geographically separated from the virus, you have little chance of catching it. Should you already be somewhere currently deemed safe, avoid travel, especially to areas that have reported infection cases. Similarly, you should avoid going out to public areas with heavy traffic whenever possible, especially if there have been cases of infection in your area. Entering into these sorts of high traffic public spaces can put you at higher risk of coming into contact with the virus. When possible, it is best to remain indoors, and get some fresh air away from other people.

If you must go out in public in an area that is known to have coronavirus cases, follow the recommendations given by healthcare professionals. In this circumstance, you may wish to wear a mask, but they are generally more effective for sick people who wish to reduce the risk of coughing or sneezing on someone else or on a surface rather than providing foolproof protection for a healthy person. When you cough or sneeze, even if you do not believe you have caught the virus, try to do so into a tissue or into the crook of your elbow with your face pointing towards the floor. This helps reduce the chances of respiratory droplets spreading to others or landing on surfaces.

Health Habits

Practicing a few easy habits that promote health and well-being can go a long way towards preventing an infection. Practicing proper hygiene does not take much time and it is well worth the marginal effort. You may have already heard people talking about handwashing as part of preventative measures. Viruses can live on the skin of your hands, picked up from public spaces and infected surfaces, and then be transferred to your eyes, nose, and mouth. This is why you should refrain from touching your face as much as possible and be sure to wash your hands before doing so. But what makes proper handwashing such an important recommendation? It has to do with the principles of virology.

As previously discussed, viruses have outer coatings that protect them and allow them to live outside of a host cell for a limited amount of time. Often these are just protein capsids, but some viruses have an additional outer envelope made out of lipids, which are fat-based. The coronavirus has this sort of layer. Soapy water breaks down fats and oils on our dishes; it can do the same to the outer lipid layer of the coronavirus. Washing your hands well with soap and water breaks down the outer envelope and, in doing so, destroys the virus. When washing your hands, you should be sure to wash for at least 20 seconds, and scrub all parts of your hands including the backs of your hands and the areas in between your fingers.

Handwashing is not the only healthy habit you should engage in. It is also a good idea to refrain from sharing food and drink with others. Eating from the same plate, using the same fork, or drinking from the same glass provides a way for the virus to transfer between people and increases the likelihood that one of you will become sick. Even if neither of you believe you have the virus, it is better to be safe and drink out of two different glasses or split the meal in half before eating rather than sharing dishware and utensils.

Supporting Your Immune System

You can also take steps to ensure your immune system is as strong as it can be. One easy way to do so is to make sure you are getting enough rest each day. Sleep deprivation can make you feel poor and put a strain on your immune system as a result. Try to get at least seven hours of sleep whenever possible so your body has the energy it needs to fight off any viruses. Regular exercise can also help increase your health as a whole.

Your diet also plays an important role in keeping you healthy. A well-balanced diet that contains plenty of vitamins and minerals supports an effective immune system. Vitamin C is one of the most critical vitamins for good immune system function. You can get vitamin C from many different fruits. Vitamin E and B6 also improve your ability to fight off or mitigate the severity of an infection. Make sure you are getting all the vitamins you need, whether through your diet or through supplements. It is also a good idea to limit the amount of alcohol you drink, as it can function as a suppressant for your immune system and make it harder for you to fight off the coronavirus should you come into contact with it.

Supply List

In many areas, people are flocking to the stores to stock their pantries in fear of an outbreak in their town and a potential quarantine. While it is a good idea to stock up on certain things, plenty of people tend to go overboard in their panic and purchase things they do not need and which will not have any impact on their continued health. Having a good idea of what purchases will be helpful and what will yield few if any benefits can help you some money and make sure you are sticking to the most effective methods of prevention and treatment.

What to Stock up On

In general, the items you may want to consider buying tend to be geared towards sanitation and disinfectant. You should have a bottle or two of hand soap, and you may also want to pick up a bottle of hand sanitizer for easy on the go use. Disinfectants can also be useful for wiping down shared spaces and ensuring that there are no viruses remaining on commonly used surfaces. If you get prescription medication, you may wish to get your next refill early if possible. This prevents you from needing to make a repeat trip and lets you spend more time at home, with the added benefit of avoiding any potential delays in medication availability.

For as many things you may want to add to your grocery list, there are just as many that there is no need to stock up on. Remember that this is a virus outbreak, not a snowstorm, and even a quarantine will not mean that you are stuck in your house without access to food and water. You may want to keep some nutritious and easy to make food on-hand just so you do not need to make a grocery run should you become ill, but you generally do not need to worry about buying a month's worth of food and water. Water especially is not a big concern; water has not been shut off in Wuhan China during the quarantine, so there is little reason to believe it will be shut off anywhere else. Tap water should be as readily available during a potential quarantine as it is now. Another popular purchase that is not as helpful as it seems is face masks. While they are good for preventing a sick person from coughing or sneezing onto others, they do very little to keep a healthy person from getting sick, and stockpiling them is not likely to help you.

The primary thing to keep in mind when buying during an outbreak is not to make panic purchases and end up with many things that you do not need. This is as true for unhelpful items as it is for buying excess quantities of even the most helpful things. While it's a good idea to keep some hand sanitizer around, there is no reason to buy an entire pallet of it. Making purchases in moderation ensures that everyone else is able to get the supplies they need to stay healthy as well, which means there are fewer sick people, which in turn means you will come in contact with the virus much less often. It is in your best interest to avoid hoarding items and allow the rest of your community to buy what they need as well, and it has the added benefit of ensuring you do not spend an entire paycheck on items you may not end up using by the end of the outbreak.

Medicine and Other Potential Treatments

Most treatments for the virus focus on minimizing the common symptoms, since there is not yet a cure for the coronavirus. Because of this, many people have begun stocking up on potential treatment methods. Unfortunately, not all available medication is helpful for the current situation, despite common misconceptions. Many people purchase antibacterial products and medications to try to keep themselves from getting sick, but the coronavirus is not a product of bacteria, so these medicines do little to affect it. This means antibiotics do not affect the virus, nor do they help treat symptoms like coughing and viral pneumonia. Make sure that any disinfectants you buy say that they are antiviral, not just antibacterial.

Some have suggested that ingesting alcohol may help fight off the virus, but virologists disagree. As mentioned previously, alcohol interferes with your body's regular immune system processes, which means that drinking is not an effective solution. It may even be putting you more at risk. Drinking plenty of water, on the other hand, prevents potential dehydration and limits the severity of fevers by helping to regulate your body's temperature.

Many treatment methods based in alternative medicine have been proposed, such as certain teas, essential oils, and herbal remedies. Unfortunately, according to experts, "There is no scientific evidence that any of these alternative remedies can prevent or cure the illness by this virus"

(NIH, 2020, para. 2). Relying on them to combat the virus and assuming their effectiveness can be dangerous, especially if they are taken in lieu of seeking medical treatment. As of now, there are no proven treatments for the coronavirus; there are only ways to moderate your symptoms.

Still, there are certain over the counter medications that may help in the case of an infection. While they may not cure the coronavirus, they can ease your symptoms and help get you back on your feet. Look for medicines that deal with the common symptoms like a persistent cough and shortness of breath. This usually means medication for cold symptoms will be helpful, as will medications that target fevers. You may want to invest in a thermometer if you do not already have one so you can identify and monitor a possible fever. If you have asthma or a similar respiratory condition, it is a good idea to keep an inhaler around as well, as the virus can make it harder for people with weaker respiratory systems to breathe.

The Coronavirus and Pets

Recently, there has been some concern over whether or not household pets can become sick with the coronavirus. We know the virus came from an animal, most likely bats, but could your cat or dog also pose a threat? Alternatively, should you be taking steps to protect your pets from the coronavirus?

The worry largely comes from a report of samples taken from one dog in Hong Kong that tested positive for the virus. Many pet owners took this as a sign that their pets may not be as safe from the virus as they had once assumed. However, there is currently no reason to believe that you can either catch or give coronavirus to your animals in the same way that it can be transmitted between humans, and "Both Hong Kong Society for the Prevention of Cruelty to Animals (SPCA) and the World Organization for Animal Health reiterated that there is no evidence of pets becoming sick with COVID-19" (Hollingsworth, 2020, para. 10). You can rest assured that your pet will not be negatively impacted by the current coronavirus outbreak.

If this is true, then how could a dog have tested positive for an infection? This is because the presence of the virus does not necessarily indicate that an animal is experiencing the same symptoms an infected human would. The coronavirus can survive on object surfaces for a certain length of time, which means "coronavirus could be present on the surface of a dog or cat, even if the dog or cat hasn't actually contracted the virus" (Hollingsworth, 2020, para. 18). Additionally, you are no more likely to catch the virus from your pet than from a rail on the subway or at a grocery store. While you should always practice proper handwashing after coming into contact with a potential infection source, there is no need to separate yourself from your pet, nor do you need to take any special precautions to keep them from getting sick.

How to Proceed If You Suspect an Infection

Due to the rapid rate of transmission of the coronavirus, there is a chance that you or a loved one may suspect you have caught the virus. If you do believe you have caught the coronavirus, the first thing to remember is don't panic. While the virus can be harmful, there are far more people who catch it and fully recover than there are who have died because of it. You most likely have a very good chance of making a complete recovery as well. The best thing you can do in this situation is have a level head, remember the facts, and take note of your symptoms. Keeping calm and proceeding rationally allows you to determine what your next move should be. Remember that there are plenty of reasons to not lose hope; to see them, you must only look at the statistics for the coronavirus.

Mortality Rate

With all of the coverage it has received, it is easy to assume that the coronavirus is a highly deadly disease. In truth, it is much less dangerous to most people than you might initially be led to believe. The most recent estimates suggest that "about 3.4% of reported COVID-19 cases have died" (WHO, 2020-d, para. 24). While this does mean that the virus can result in death, it also means that currently, the overwhelming majority of people who develop symptoms of the virus do not die. In fact, the number may even be lower than the suggested 3.4%, as that number only takes into account the results of reported cases. There are likely many more people who have recovered and have had mild enough symptoms that they did not think to contact a doctor, or people who were treated without the infection being reported to the World Health Organization (WHO). There is no reason to assume that simply contracting the virus means you will not survive, even if you have a lowered immune system or your age puts you at a greater risk. Many people in these same conditions have made recoveries, and you have every reason to believe that you will too.

Your Next Steps

You may be tempted to rush out to the nearest doctor's office or hospital waiting room and get treatment at the first sign of a light cough, but experts actually recommend that most people who catch the coronavirus remain at home. This is of course dependent on the severity of your symptoms. If you are experiencing nothing worse than average cold symptoms, you likely do not need to seek immediate medical attention. A few days of bedrest and relaxation may be all you need to feel better. Like with any cold or flu virus, if you feel sick, you should take time off from work or school and stay home. Trying to continue to work as usual, or sitting in a hospital waiting room, brings you into contact with more people and increases the chances that you will spread the virus to others. People in hospital waiting rooms may have a harder time fighting off a viral infection due to the illness or injury they came to the hospital to treat, so they are especially vulnerable.

If your symptoms worsen and you start to suspect you will no longer be able to take care of yourself, you should then seek medical treatment. If possible, call ahead to local treatment centers and schedule an appointment; this reduces the time you have to spend out of the house and around others in a waiting room where you might spread the virus. Many towns, businesses, and universities have established their own protocols to follow to report a potential case of coronavirus, so be sure to check the ones that apply to you. A school may need to know about a new case, even a mild one, so they can take steps to protect other students; many businesses have decided to follow a similar practice. Proper communication can help to prevent a local outbreak.

Finally, do not lose faith that you will recover. The mortality rate for the virus is still very low, and there is little indication that it will raise in the near future. Believing that you will feel better can be a powerful force that can contribute to your recovery, as it encourages you to actively pursue routes of treatment. With enough rest, fluids, and medical aid if necessary, you are very likely to be back on your feet in no time.

Chapter 2: Myths and Misunderstandings

Due to the widespread coverage the coronavirus has received, there is a lot of room for error. When everyone is trying to get out information as quickly as possible, some news becomes outdated just as quickly as it is released, while other information falls through the cracks for a variety of reasons. Additionally, with so many people affected, there are sure to be a large number of perspectives and viewpoints on the issue. All of this coverage and debate can produce misinformation, intentional or otherwise, that leads to fear and panic. The WHO has gone as far as to refer to the situation as an "infodemic," which they describe as "an over-abundance of information — some accurate and some not — that makes it hard for people to find trustworthy sources and reliable guidance when they need it" (WHO, 2020, para. 5). This is a serious concern for people who want to know what they should be doing and what to look out for during an outbreak.

There are many commonly believed myths about the coronavirus that have achieved wide circulation at some point during coverage. Many of them come from the early days of the virus when there was less available information or statistics were different from what they are now. Others are a result of conspiracy theories, stereotypes, and incorrect assumptions. Some of them come from news outlets that simply want to drive views and lean towards more provocative and sensationalist headlines to do so, or from governments that want to reassure their citizens but do so by potentially minimizing the effect the virus has had in their country. Despite any possible good intentions, myths about the coronavirus can leave the public less informed, lead them to unknowingly make poor decisions that may put them at higher risk of getting sick, and interfere with efforts to stop the spread of the coronavirus. Debunking these myths and examining other potential sources of misinformation will help you separate the facts from the fabrications.

Fact Checking Common Rumors

Some of the most common rumors and myths can be debunked through simple fact checking. Others require a slightly complicated explanation to identify the truth. Examining each rumor in detail sheds light on possible sources of misunderstanding.

Face Masks

Face masks have been one of the most hoarded items since the outbreak began. People have flocked to stores buying up stacks of masks, believing them to be an effective deterrent of catching the virus. Many people assume that wearing a face mask when they go out will keep them healthy. Despite this common assumption, are face masks really as helpful for most people as the rush to buy them would lead you to believe?

The short answer is no. Though face masks are useful for healthy people in some situations, they are not especially useful for the average person. Face masks will help to keep someone sick from spreading the illness through coughing or sneezing, but they do not do much for healthy people wearing them and have not been linked to lower levels of viral infection. You do not need to rush out to the store to buy a mask or pay double the price to get one from a reseller now that they are being hoarded; you are better off just washing your hands frequently and avoiding touching your face.

Though most people will get little to no benefit from masks, there are some situations in which masks may actually help you. This is primarily true for health care workers who will come into close contact with multiple sick patients, or for others who are acting as caregivers to sick friends or relatives. Buying mass amounts of face masks if you are not in one of these situations can make it harder for those who need them to access them. This can lead to doctors and other health providers getting sick and leaving fewer people available to treat the virus, so dispelling the myth about face masks goes a long way towards improving public health as a whole.

Ethnic Profiling

The spread of the coronavirus has led to a number of harmful stereotypes about those living in infected areas. Some people have targeted people from China or anyone of Asian descent, incorrectly assuming that they must be carrying the virus. This is especially true for Asian-Americans, many of whom may not have even left the country during the time of the outbreak. Some have even assumed that people from China are more susceptible to infection, more likely to be the source of an infection, and are more likely to be carriers, even though China is far from the only country to be infected.

These rumors are not just harmful to those being targeted, but also to those spreading them. The truth is that the coronavirus does not discriminate based on nationality or ethnicity, and those who assume it does can actually end up making themselves more vulnerable to the virus due to their misinformation. Building a culture of shame around the virus discourages people from seeking medical treatment when they need it and keeps them from taking proper health precautions. Decreasing the stigma around the coronavirus encourages people to get the help they need and keeps all of us safer.

Man-Made Origins

Since the beginning of the virus, rumors have circulated about its origination, especially before researchers identified a likely cause. Some theorized that the virus was not a product of nature but instead a result of lab testing. The most popular rumors seem to indicate that the coronavirus was created in a research lab in China and escaped to infect the public. Some other rumors have suggested that the virus was made in other countries and was carried to China, whether inadvertently or as a purposeful act that got out of hand.

These rumors are little more than conspiracy theories. The most likely source of the virus is from bats or another animal, not from any man-made sources. There is no evidence to suggest that the virus was created on purpose, and all available evidence and previous experiences with coronaviruses points towards an animal source. Myths of a deadly virus of our own making only serve to breed fear and distrust, which interferes with prevention and treatment.

Home Treatments

All manner of possible solutions have come from various sources during the outbreak. Some claim that buying a certain miracle product can prevent infection and destroy existing infections, while others suggest you use household items to fight off the virus. The types of possible treatments vary greatly and include medicinal herbs, foods and drinks, ingesting silver, drinking alcohol, and many others. Some have even suggested using bleach to 'disinfect' your skin or, worse, ingesting bleach and other cleaning products.

It is clear that drinking harmful chemicals, even heavily diluted, will not improve your overall health, and it will do nothing to improve your immunity against the virus. Some of the other methods may initially seem plausible, but they are quickly disproven. There are currently no approved cures for the coronavirus, which means that everything from essential oils to bottles of high-proof vodka will be ineffective and potentially dangerous, especially if they replace more conventional symptom treatment methods. Home treatments should be approached with suspicion; while they may sound like amazing methods for staying safe at first glance, their effectiveness ranges from little to no difference to actively harmful. Until a cure is approved by official sources, you should stay away from anything claiming to cure the coronavirus.

Infected Packages

Some people have wondered if ordering shipments from countries where there have been many cases of infection is a wise move. The thought process is that should someone who is sick come into contact with your package, the virus might travel through the shipping process and arrive at your door along with your purchase. This has made people hesitant to purchase products from overseas, even if previously they did not feel any need to be cautious.

Luckily, packages sent through the mail do not seem to be capable of transmitting the virus to you. Though the coronavirus can survive on surfaces for a given length of time, it does not seem to be capable of surviving a journey that spans multiple days. By the time a package or envelope reaches you, the virus will not have survived the trip and you can open your packages without any worry. The only source of concern may come in the form of delays caused by a weakened workforce and quarantines. These can slow supply chains and interfere with the timeliness of your purchases, but this is an unavoidable concern in an outbreak situation, especially one that involves such a large exporter of goods like China.

Heat Sensitivity

Cold and flu viruses tend to be more prevalent in the colder months. This has led many to believe that as the warmer months approach, the coronavirus will simply disappear. The coronavirus may be heat sensitive, and once the spring arrives the number of cases should plummet accordingly, turning the virus into something we either only have to deal with seasonally or ending it altogether.

While this is a nice idea, it is currently impossible to know whether or not warmer weather will have any impact on the coronavirus. We do not yet know enough about this strain of coronavirus to know if warm weather creates sub-optimal replication conditions or if the virus is aided by colder temperatures at all. Additionally, there are many different theories as to why cold and flu viruses are less prevalent in the summer months, and not all of them suggest that warm weather itself is the culprit. For example, something like more time spent indoors and sharing germs with others in the winter may contribute. Either way, it is very unlikely that the arrival of spring will simply cause all cases of the virus to disappear. It is also not strictly true that similar diseases only circulate in the colder months; while the cold may act as an immune system suppressant and leave us more susceptible to infection, this does not mean that we are completely immune as soon as it hits 70 degrees. The SARS outbreak of 2003 did not report its last cases until July, which is well into the summer. Since both are coronaviruses, the chances of COVID-19 being especially sensitive to higher temperatures seems unlikely at present, though only time will tell.

Suspicions of Under-Reporting

Some people have claimed that certain countries are under-reporting the number of coronavirus cases they have dealt with since the beginning of the outbreak. These accusations usually center around China and come from both sources inside China, such as citizens who live in Wuhan and don't believe the extent of the outbreak is being accurately portrayed, and sources outside of China, such as reporters and some health officials who are dubious about the number of claims.

China in particular is in a difficult situation with the current coronavirus outbreak, being the country of origin and facing a lot of pressure to manage the situation before it can get worse. This is why many believe they have been greatly underestimating the number of cases and failing to relay those that are reported to them by different provinces. Theoretically, if China reports lower numbers, it will appear as though the disease is under control. Fewer people getting sick means the virus is being successfully contained, which looks much better for both China and the rest of the world as it suggests that the right measures are being taken to combat the virus. Unfortunately, the doubt that these lower numbers are really true has impeded upon public faith in their government organizations and the governments of other countries to adequately handle the disease and provide us with correct information.

China is not the only country to be suspected of fudging the numbers. Other nations have also come under accusations recently, especially those that are currently experiencing large scale outbreaks. One such nation is Iran, where "Iranian members of parliament and health officials allege that the government is grossly under-reporting the death toll as well as the spread of the disease to the public" (Keyser, 2020, para. 4). Concerns of misrepresented numbers are a global issue. Every country has the opportunity to fail to report cases, just as every country has the opportunity to be accurate and transparent with its citizens and the rest of the world.

But is there any truth to these rumors? How certain can we be that numbers are being under-reported, and what does it mean if they are?

To tackle only the question of the truthfulness of this rumor, it is hard to say at the current time. Since each nation's government provides the only verified source of infection and death reports, it is not easy to compare the number of reported cases with how many are actually occurring. A firm answer one way or another would likely be dependent on being physically present in the affected countries, observing the number of cases, and collecting data directly from hospitals, but as this carries with it a high risk of infection, it is unlikely that such a count will take place any time soon. Just as people have claimed under-reporting, so too have people claimed that there is likely nothing insidious about the current virus numbers that would suggest any cover-up attempts. This has led many to question that, if we assume understated reports are being presented, are the numbers being under-reported purposefully or is there more to the situation?

Purposeful or Incidental

Many people believe that not only are the numbers being falsified, but that this is being done on purpose in an attempt to quell public panic. However, some have countered that the lower than expected numbers may not actually be a deliberate choice on any government's part but simply an incidental result of nearly all outbreaks. The differences in what is seen and what is reported may simply be a product of limited data that does not account for everyone who has fallen ill.

The theory of incidental under-reporting claims that the majority of cases being reported are those that showcase more severe symptoms. People who end up in hospitals are more likely to be those who need critical care rather than those likely to make a full recovery. In the wake of allegations of China purposefully faking numbers, "experts were quick to note that the Chinese are not willfully underreporting cases," instead pointing out that "when thousands of sick people show up at hospitals looking for care, there is no time to go searching for people who have mild symptoms and who have stayed home" (Branswell, 2020, para. 3). Additionally, when there is so much do it in terms of medical care, policy recommendations, and research, reporting new cases is not always the first thing on anyone's mind. It is possible that in all of the pandemonium, a certain number of cases have been skipped over, even if they were reported by hospitals or other care facilities. If you add this to the fact that those with very mild symptoms do not tend to go to the doctor at all, and instead are being encouraged to remain at home unless their symptoms progress, this means even fewer people with mild versions of the illness are being counted. All of this can lead to artificially inflated death rates and ideas about how severe the illness is, as only those who are the most sick are being counted.

This evidence seems to suggest that while under-reporting may be occurring, it is most likely not being done as an active cover-up of the extent and severity of the virus; on the contrary, lower numbers of reported cases compared to those that led to deaths may actually be making the death rate seem worse than it is. Unfortunately, misinformation and uncertainty created by the idea of under-reported cases can harm public opinion, whether it is being done purposefully or otherwise.

What's the Difference?

The matter of under-reporting infection numbers is bigger than just a few cases that may have slipped through the cracks. The existence of a possible issue being brought to public attention has serious ramifications, whether it is eventually proven true or false. While the possibility that the mortality rate is actually lower than what has been calculated with our current numbers is definitely a good thing, this does not mean that the idea of the virus' damage being covered up, even accidentally, sits well with most people. Many will hear that the virus is being under-reported and immediately enter into panic, assuming the infection rate and death toll must then be something worth covering up. This can lead to a great deal of panic and fear.

These rumors also undermine public trust in world leadership, which can make it harder to deliver important health and safety information in the future. If people do not think they can trust their government for clear, accurate information, this uncertainty does not go away so easily. People may then proceed to ignore recommendations to remain indoors, avoid travel, and take washing their hands seriously because they have lost faith in the accuracy of all information being delivered to them.

Artificially lowered reports can also lead to problems as the virus continues to spread in different countries across the globe. If other countries do not see the virus as a threat and take its spread seriously, they may not make the appropriate preparations. This can lead to inadequate containment methods and a lack of public education, which can ultimately provide the virus with a foothold in a new country. As an example, many countries hesitated to instate travel quarantines on those who had come from countries with the virus because it was not believed to be as prevalent. Once the numbers began to increase, temporary quarantines and tests after travel were put into place, but anyone who came off a plane carrying the virus had likely already infected a number of people. Under-reporting can lead people to believe the virus is not something to be worried about and let their guard down just as much as it can inspire panic over the virus. In either case, the virus benefits while people are left uninformed and uncertain of their next action.

It is incredibly important for reports of coronavirus infections and deaths to be accurate. Without accuracy, proper containment methods may be viewed as unnecessary and, once the difference in case numbers is discovered, people may stop trusting certain sources of information. Whether the potential discrepancy is purposeful or due to unforeseen errors, it still has an impact on public opinion and actions.

Public Health Emergency

On January 30th, 2020, the WHO announced that the coronavirus outbreak had ushered us into a Public Health Emergency of International Concern (PHEIC). This announcement made many people understandably concerned. It seemed to suggest the virus was a very big threat, and had many believing that the coronavirus would be the next big plague that wiped us all out. Those who did not immediately assume the worst were still largely uncertain as to what the declaration of a public health emergency meant. What exactly does such a designation imply, and how does it change how official organizations are already attempting to tackle the coronavirus?

What Is a Global Public Health Emergency?

A PHEIC is a health concern that has become a global problem. It is something that the rest of the world should watch out for, even if it has not yet been sighted in every country. It generally suggests that a solution to the current problem would require a shared effort and cooperation between countries, whether this comes in the form of research or relief efforts. It does not always have to be a virus; it may also indicate another source of illness, such as a dangerous chemical accidentally released into close contact with people or purposefully used as a form of chemical warfare. It may also apply to certain nuclear radiation situations.

What a PHEIC does not necessarily mean is that we have entered a pandemic situation, as that status only came much later for the coronavirus, nor does it mean that there is any reason to panic and assume death is imminent. Many PHEIC declarations serve to inform global governments that a potential threat is on its way, but they do not necessarily imply that the threat is especially severe compared to past public health emergencies. For example, new strains of influenza are automatically added to the list of public health emergencies, regardless of whether or not their mortality rates are higher or lower than existing strains. Other emergencies that did not need an official declaration to be added to the PHEIC registry are polio, SARS, and smallpox. Since the designation was not formally introduced until 2005 as a result of the SARS epidemic, many of these diseases occurred before the naming convention existed, though any new strains and cases would still be regarded as PHEICs.

Though there are quite a few diseases that automatically get designated as global emergencies, there have been relatively few actual declarations of PHEIC outside of these automatic cases. The 2009 H1N1 was the first, and the current coronavirus outbreak is the most recent. Other examples include the 2014 Ebola outbreak, the 2015 concerns over the Zika virus, and the still ongoing Kivu Ebola outbreak which began in 2018. COVID-19 is only the sixth time that a PHEIC has been formally declared.

Why Was the Coronavirus Named a Global Concern?

Presently, it is easy to see why the coronavirus is a problem for everyone, not just China. The virus has already spread to many different countries, and it may continue to spread to more. However, back in January the virus did not seem like it was going to become such a widespread problem. It was not just a problem for China, of course, but it did not have nearly the same global reach as it does currently. Despite this, the WHO was quick to name the outbreak a PHEIC and encourage global support for affected nations in containing the coronavirus' spread. Why, if the virus was not yet present in so many countries, did it become a worldwide problem so quickly?

The answer does not involve a conspiracy theory about a cover-up of early contagion cases outside of China, nor does it involve any sort of ulterior motives as some have suggested. Instead, it was an effort to increase global awareness and support as well as an attempt to prevent further spread of the virus. In the statement that declared the coronavirus a PHEIC, the WHO said the new categorization was performed "in the spirit of support and appreciation for China, its people, and the actions China has taken on the frontlines of this outbreak," as well as the feeling that "a global coordinated effort is needed to enhance preparedness in other regions of the world that may need additional support" (WHO, 2020, para. 17). By making the coronavirus a global issue, the WHO sought to encourage people from all nations to consider the likelihood that it may come to their country, which in turn would spur them to lend their knowledge and resources to the effort to fight the virus.

The declaration of a public health emergency has already aided with relief efforts, even as the virus has continued to spread since the end of January. Countries are better prepared for possible cases of the coronavirus and quarantine measures for travelers are more common. Additionally, strategies for possible treatments are being examined in multiple countries. While it is unlikely that we will see a COVID-19 vaccine any time soon, further research and the development of reliable diagnosis and care strategies has been greatly expedited by so many people coming together to help end the virus' spread. PHEIC declarations encourage minds from all across the globe to lend their aid to the project to keep everyone safer and helps unite people during what could otherwise be a very divisive time. Though a public health emergency may sound frightening at first, it is actually a step in the right direction for preventing the coronavirus outbreak from becoming a more serious concern.

Use of Drone Technology

Technological advancements have played a role in the way China is responding to the coronavirus. New devices that have been employed to fight the virus include artificial intelligence programs and remotely controlled drones. This may sound like a strange, somewhat dystopian development, and many have taken it to mean such. It is a bit hard to picture a drone coming to your door and delivering food while you are on lockdown and not also imagine any number of worrying implications. Comparisons to everything from *I, Robot* to *1984* have surfaced, largely led by confused onlookers that could not imagine seeing these developments in their own towns. But is this implementation of tech to fight off the virus a cause for concern, or just a unique use of resources to fight a mounting problem?

Though the idea may sound foreign to many people, there are benefits to the concept. For one, robots cannot get sick like humans can, so using them in place of human contact helps to limit the potential for the virus to spread. While humans must interact with these robots at some point, they are more easily disinfected and wiped down of any lingering viruses than people, so there is less chance of them accidentally helping to spread the coronavirus.

Robots and drones are most commonly being used to limit the amount of human to human contact during the outbreak. They can facilitate conversation between patients and doctors without needing to expose doctors to a potential infection for longer than is necessary. They are also being used as delivery services, both for those stuck in their homes and in public. Delivery of food and supplies has been made much easier thanks to technology, as they can be sent to houses to deliver goods or sent to hospitals and clinics to provide new medical supplies. Some restaurants have even adopted the use of delivery robots to bring food out to customers, reducing the risk of transferring disease between patrons and staff. Other robots and drones have been used for disinfection purposes, able to safely patrol the halls and rooms of hospitals without putting janitorial staff at risk. Additionally, supercomputers capable of running incredibly quick calculations and tests have been used to speed up research towards a cure. Most of these methods seem relatively harmless in practice if a little isolating, but one use of drones that has drawn some controversy is using technology to look for people in need of treatment. This most commonly involves temperature scanners that can locate people with fevers, but the same drones can also be used to ensure people are complying with any quarantine rules that have been set.

Any use of technology for surveillance, whether for diagnosis or patrol, carries with it some potential for misuse. There is an inherent loss of personal privacy for people already in a difficult situation. There is also not much opportunity for people to opt out of this increased surveillance. While ending the spread of the virus is important, it is also important to keep privacy concerns in mind; tech that oversteps its boundaries may be met with hostility rather than cooperation, which can interfere with efforts to contain COVID-19.

Chapter 3: Wuhan China

Most people only know Wuhan from the coverage of the coronavirus. If you do not live in China, it is very likely that you have never heard of the location before. This means that the only picture you have in your mind of the area is what you have learned on the news about the virus. It can seem very foreign, both literally and metaphorically, from your own town. Wuhan's notoriety is an unfortunate consequence of its role as the epicenter of the coronavirus, but boiling it down to just what has been said in the media is doing the city a great disservice.

Wuhan is much more than just a point of origin for COVID-19. It is a thriving city that is home to great numbers of people who, prior to the infection, lived busy and highly varied lives. It is a hub of parks, commercial life, sprawling lakes, and historical sites that make it much more than just a city impacted by illness and locked into quarantine. It can be easy to simply view it in the abstract sense, but recognizing that Wuhan is full of life and people helps to humanize it in our minds. Wuhan may be half a world away from you or it may be right next door, but it shares many similarities with many of the world's largest cities, all with its own unique culture and lifestyle. Just as the WHO's declaration of the coronavirus as a global emergency spurred people from all walks of life to action, having a better understanding of what the city of Wuhan was like before the virus hit can encourage us to lend our own support to those who have been hit the hardest by COVID-19.

Wuhan Before the Outbreak

Before people were encouraged to remain indoors and avoid extended contact with others, Wuhan was an extremely large, bustling city. It is located in the Hubei province in China, and it serves as the province's capital city. It is also the largest city in Hubei and has the highest population of a single city within Central China. Because of this, it is home to many companies and businesses as well as a great deal of people. Wuhan houses over 11 million people on a daily basis. To put this number into perspective, this is nearly 1.5 times the population of big cities like New York City and London, and nearly four times the population of Los Angeles. To say that Wuhan is a big city is certainly an understatement, and to say it is a busy one is a similarly reserved description of the sheer amount of activity that occurs within Wuhan.

Thanks in part to its size, Wuhan is a center of development for China. It has a strong focus on education, politics, the economy, and manufacturing. It is home to a number of large businesses that engage in nation-wide trade such as Dongfeng Motor Corporation, which produces cars and other automotive vehicles, and Biolake, which is a bioindustry base involved in the research and production of pharmaceutical and medical biotechnology. The city is also home to the largest power production station in the world, the Three Gorges Dam, which is fueled by the Yangtze River. The education focus in Wuhan can be seen through the presence of many schools and colleges. Both the Huazhong University of

Science and Technology and Wuhan University provide higher education to Chinese residents and international students alike.

Wuhan is also benefitted by its many avenues of transportation. It is full of roads, train railways, and express highways that keep it connected to its neighbors and ensure a frequent inflow of new visitors every day. Unfortunately, the city's role as a hub of transportation may have inadvertently made it easier for the coronavirus to spread to other provinces and even to other countries. Still, outside of recent events, Wuhan's connection to other cities and nations has made it an intricate and diverse meeting of many different cultures and ideas.

Tourism

Wuhan is not just a home to its residents but also a temporary home to many travelers. Its ties to tourism are very strong, and every year thousands of visitors from all across the globe come to the city. The city boasts a wide variety of attractions, both cutting edge and ancient; new businesses line the streets, carefully arranged alongside historic sites connected to previous uprisings and political movements in the city's history. One of the biggest tourist attractions is the Yellow Crane Tower, which dates back to as early as 200 AD, and has weathered many destruction attempts and rebuilding since then. It is a staggeringly high tower on the Yangtze River with connections to ancient legends and the practice of Taoism, making it a popular tourist destination. Other historical sites include memorials and temples.

Wuhan also contains plenty of parks and other outdoor areas. There is a large botanical garden with thousands of different species of plants and greenery. There are also many lakes within and nearby the city. Wuhan is home to a number of different markets, each boasting a wide variety of souvenirs and essential goods alike. The Wuhan Zoo has tigers, monkeys, and of course, pandas. Wuhan even contains a theme park that is a host to many carnival-style rides and games. Visitors to the city have plenty to do to pack their trips with both enjoyment and education.

Culture

Wuhan is also a huge cultural hub. It is regarded as one of the origin points of Chu culture in ancient China. Chu was one of the largest countries in the Hubei province during its zenith, and Chu culture refers to the deep history of both the Chu state and the Chu clan. It was an extremely powerful state that produced plenty of relics and artifacts that are still on display in Wuhan to this day. Chu fabrics, especially those crafted from silk, remain popular, as do bronze castings, many of which are thousands of years old.

The city is also home to many stages and opera houses in the style of Han opera, a traditional style that has maintained popularity around the Yangtze River area. It remains the most common type of opera performed within Wuhan, and locals and travelers alike often come to Wuhan to watch performances.

One of Wuhan's primary cultural sites is the Ancient Lute Platform, which has connections to ancient folklore. According to legends, it is the central location of the well-known story of Yu Boya and Zhong Ziqi, which is considered part of China's National Intangible Cultural Heritage. The story is representative of close friendship, as in it, the musician Boya plays his guqin for an onlooker, Ziqi, and declares Ziqi is the only one who truly understands his music (Government of Hubei, 2014, para. 6). The Lute Platform is said to be the spot where Boya played his melodies in the tale. Since 2011, the Lute Platform has been the home to annual musical competitions that carry on the spirit of the ancient folktale.

Wuhan's music ties are not just relegated to ancient times. More modern musical movements have found a home in Wuhan as well. This is especially true of punk music, which has strong ties to the area. Wuhan is also associated with many local foods, specifically hot and dry noodles, which the city has become famous for. Both of these cultural touchstones will be discussed in further detail shortly. Though Wuhan has many modern influences, it is also a city defined by its rich history.

A Brief History

Wuhan is a city that holds great historical significance and has been the site of many important events. While today there are a great deal of modern technological advancements and cutting-edge businesses to be seen in the city, they are integrated with the ancient aspects to form a more cohesive whole that tells the complete history of the area. The city has been an area of great prosperity and industry for generations, which is a tradition that still continues on today. Looking further back into its history reveals the role it played in big historical events such as revolutions and political upheavals.

Founding

Wuhan was formed through the merging of three already existing towns along the Han and Yangtze River, specifically where the two rivers met. These were the towns of Wuchang, located on the Yangtze's southern bank; Hankou, situated on the north bank of the two rivers; and Hanyang, which sat between the two rivers near where they intersected. Each of these towns had their own distinct qualities and cultures that influenced the sort of city Wuhan became after the merge.

The town of Wuchang once functioned as the capital of the province during the Yuan dynasty. As a result, it had become a center for education and the arts, housing many scholars and their students. Hankou, on the other hand, was more involved in economics and trade. It was briefly invaded by the British during the mid-1800s and used as a large trading port, and even after the British no longer controlled the area, it remained one of the largest economic areas in China for many years. Hanyang was and is still a largely industrial area.

The three cities were not merged until 1926, when a military campaign known as the Northern Expedition decided it should become the new capital city of Nationalist China. This was a product of the Chinese

Revolution, during which the imperial dynasties were overthrown and the Republic of China was established. From then on, the large area went by the name of Wuhan, an amalgamation of 'Wu' from Wuchang and 'han' from Hanyang which formed its northern and southern borders.

The Capital City

Wuhan's role as a capital city was ushered in following the end of the Qing dynasty. Previously, the area was hotly contested between Qing and rebel forces, but after the success of the Wuchang Uprising and Xinhai Revolution that overthrew Qing reign, the Republic of China laid claim to the land. In 1927, it was declared the new capital of China by the Kuomintang (KMT) government, though this was short-lived. The capital quickly moved, but Wuhan remained a powerful, united city that spanned many miles and held just as many residents.

The 1931 China floods of the Yangtze and Huai Rivers which occurred shortly after heavily impacted Wuhan due to its location on the Yangtze. At first, Wuhan served as a refuge for many people in surrounding areas whose homes had been flooded and livelihoods destroyed, but soon it fell victim to the flooding rivers as well. Many were injured, thousands lost their homes, and the floods led to many deaths as well. These floods are seen as the worst in Chinese history, but other floods have followed. In 1936, the city was impacted by floods once more, and overflowing rivers have continued to be a severe problem for the city as recently as 2016 despite attempts to prevent the issue.

Wuhan became a capital city once more in 1937 for another brief period, this time just ten months. It was considered a wartime capital, as China was engaged in the Second Sino-Japanese War. It was temporarily controlled by Japan and served as a logistics center during this time. It would not return to Chinese control until 1945, after the end of the Second World War.

Currently, Wuhan is the capital city of just the Hubei province, not of all of China. However, its historical ties as a noteworthy city that has often been at the center of political and industrial developments can still be seen today throughout the city.

Destruction and Rebuilding

Wuhan has been subject to destruction from both natural disasters and wartime conflicts. Floods have been an issue as previously mentioned, but so have wars and other military conflicts. One of the most serious attacks occurred during World War II, when Wuhan was under Japanese control. At the time, the US was fighting against Japan, and they chose Wuhan as one of their targets. In December of 1944, "nearly 200 American planes raided the Chinese city of Wuhan, dropping 500 tons of incendiary bombs" (Harmsen, 2015, para. 1). The damage done to the city was great, with many structures being destroyed and many people injured or killed. However, after the war, Wuhan returned to Chinese control, and rebuilding efforts began. Wuhan continued to be the site of many dangerous conflicts and disasters, including the Yangtze River Floods in 1954, a fight for control of the city dubbed the Wuhan Incident, and further large flood incidents in 2010, 2011, and 2016.

Despite the somewhat turbulent times the city has experienced, each time it has been rebuilt better and stronger than before. The Three Gorges Dam, constructed to reduce the risk of flooding, has helped to limit the number of deaths resulting from major floods. The Yellow Crane Tower has been rebuilt multiple times and now stands firm as a monument and a popular tourist destination. Though the threats to the city's continued existence have been great, its continued prosperity and the sheer number of people who still call it home speaks volumes to the resilience of Wuhan for thousands of years. Many residents have looked back at these times of hardship for strength during the current outbreak, hoping that like the past, their own current situation will eventually come to an end and the city will remain a home to so many.

A City of Protest and Social Change

Wuhan has often been the site of political and social protests. Considering its connections to the Chinese Revolution, it is perhaps unsurprising that the same tradition of revolt and pushing for better conditions has continued on to this day. Protests occurred in solidarity with the Tiananmen Square protests in 1989 in the form of a railway sit-in, largely organized by students and other young activists. Two decades later, protests again erupted against the French-owned store Carrefour, which had been accused of perpetrating anti-Chinese stereotypes and sentiments. Wuhan was joined by a number of Chinese cities including Qingdao, Beijing, and Hefei. Notable protests occurred as recently as 2019, when residents discouraged the construction of a new incinerator. Wuhan continues to be a hub for social and political movements and its residents continue to band together during tough times, which can be seen during the current outbreak as well.

Even as the coronavirus continues to affect the people of Wuhan, many have refused to give up hope. It is a difficult time and it will continue to be one for the extent of the virus' life, but the city's residents are doing all they can to make the best of a bad situation. Residents have reported that, "One night, in an expression of solidarity or perhaps boredom, many decided to chant together out of their windows." During this event, "People were howling into the night sky, singing patriotic songs and calling out to support one another" (Yu, 2020, para. 27). The situation is dire, but people in Wuhan are banding together to weather the storm, just as they have banded together in previous incidents. Despite the quarantine enforcing physical separation, community remains as important to Wuhan residents as it does for so many of us. This is perhaps one of the reasons why recognition of the cultural touchstones of Wuhan, such as local dishes and art movements, is so important.

Wuhan Noodles

Wuhan has plenty of unique dishes enjoyed by locals and tourists alike. It is especially well-known for Wuhan noodles, also known as hot and dry noodles and locally as reganmian. The name refers to the texture of the noodles, which are favored with sesame paste, giving them the somewhat dry taste while still packing a punch. Wuhan noodles are considered one of the most famous Chinese noodle dishes, and generally rank very favorably in terms of taste. They are made from alkaline noodles, frequently also used in ramen dishes, which are made with the addition of sodium carbonate to make them less acidic than standard noodles. Most recipes include sesame paste, sesame oil, garlic, soy sauce, and other spices to add heat. Some add sides or toppings of green onion, pickled radish, or pickled green beans. Depending on taste preferences, sugar may also be added to the sauce, adding sweetness to balance the spice.

Wuhan noodles are often considered street food, and they are available year round from both street vendors and restaurants.

However, they are most commonly enjoyed during celebrations, especially during the Chinese New Year. Since many people born in China return home to celebrate the New Year, the holiday has become conflated with the meal in the city of Wuhan, and many people look forward to it as part of their festivities. They are usually eaten for breakfast, though they are often served during the rest of the day, especially in Chinese restaurants located outside of China.

Outside of the city, the rest of China strongly associates Wuhan with its noodles, the same way people in the US might associate Maine with lobster rolls or New England with clam chowder. While you can certainly order the dish outside of Wuhan or make it yourself with the right ingredients, most people agree that the city is the only way to get the most authentic dish. Prior to the onset of the coronavirus, these noodles helped to put Wuhan on the map and in the minds of residents of other Chinese provinces. Because of this, the noodles have become a way to show support for Wuhan during the outbreak and quarantine. For those outside the city looking to wish residents well any way they can, "eating hot dry noodles has become a symbol of solidarity with Wuhan and its people" (Levitt, 2020, para. 3). A number of photos and drawings created recently depict people eating Wuhan noodles. While these people may not be able to end the spread of the virus and develop an immediate cure, they can still show their concern and well wishes in this way.

Wuhan Punk

Food is not all that Wuhan's cultural scene has to offer. It is also rich with music of all kinds. Given Wuhan's connections to revolutionary movements, it is maybe no surprise that one of the most popular genres is punk. The punk movement has long since been associated with pushes for social change and anti-establishment sentiments, which have run strong in Wuhan since its inception. Punk music is a language of rebellion, resistance, and change, often associated with youth culture. In a country like China, which has often been criticized for taking steps to limit the spread of certain information or keeping an eye on what members of the public are up to, especially online, punk has found a home in the CDs and playlists of those who want to see something change.

The Chinese punk movement found purchase in Wuhan in the 1990s, largely through a number of underground bands that gained surprising popularity in the area. Beijing was another center of punk in China that allowed the music to gain more recognition despite discouragement from local and national governments. Both cities' punk movements appeared shortly after the decline of rock'n'roll, and the official location of the beginning of Chinese punk is heavily debated between the two cities. Rather than more traditional concerts, CD Bars hosted small gatherings where punk musicians would play away from the eyes of authorities, and eventually many founded private venues of their own. In Wuhan especially, the punk subculture dealt heavily with political change rather than simply being a clothing style or music genre. People in Wuhan desired change, and punk music was the avenue by which they shared their desire for it to happen.

A great deal of the punk music produced dealt with more sensitive, taboo topics that were not acceptable to broach in other genres. Political stances were common, almost expected, especially those that were critical of the government and police. In the songs and in the singers' everyday lives, "Wuhan punks often show their affection for the city, but also their aversion to a municipal government that tries to suppress every inch of popular autonomy" (Amar, 2020, para. 16). They often focus on fighting corruption, pushing back against certain legislation, and general discontent with the current state of things.

Like Wuhan noodles, punk music and the punk subculture has also become a symbol of solidarity during Wuhan's coronavirus outbreak. There have been pusbacks against the Chinese government for the suspicions of under-reporting virus cases as mentioned previously, and also for concerns that the virus was not reported right away, which may have led to many more infections and resulting deaths. These ideas have again inspired notions of rebellion in Wuhan residents, many of whom feel like they have been mistreated or that their government is not doing enough to keep people safe; prolonged surveillance and quarantine has produced a similar sentiment for many others.

Perhaps more than just rebellion, Wuhan punk music has also become a representation of resistance and resilience in the face of a threat as frightening as the coronavirus. Amidst accusations of mishandling of the virus and fears about its spread, the resilient spirit of Wuhan punk lives on in its people, encouraging them to fight off the illness and make full recoveries. Residents are making efforts to resist illness, keep themselves safe, and eventually see the end of the coronavirus.

Chapter 4: The Coronavirus Timeline

The coronavirus began in late December of 2019, but it did not become a matter of public concern and news coverage until well into January. As a result, it can be hard to fully understand the development and spread of the virus so far. A timeline helps us break down our many questions into more manageable chunks while also showing us the general progression of infection cases, as well as what governments and individuals have done in an attempt to lower the numbers. Looking back at the virus' inception in December answers questions about when exactly the virus began, what the initial spread looked like, and what initial measures were taken or failed to be taken. January and February give us an idea of how the virus spread widely enough that it started to be considered a global threat. They also show how foreign governments reacted to the possible presence of the virus. March provides the most recently available data and shows us what the current state of things are, as well as what we may need to do to ensure the infection does not continue to spread.

Having a good idea of the history of the coronavirus provides us with insights and educated guesses as to how it will continue to spread. From only our own perspectives, it is hard to know if we will see an end to this sickness soon or if it will continue on for the next few months or even years, but getting a big picture of how things have developed since December can shed some light on how much longer we may continue to encounter disturbances due to the threat of infection. While no one can know for sure what the future will hold, understanding the past helps us make predictions and contextualize the presence of the coronavirus in our own lives.

December 2019

Very little was known about the coronavirus during the month of its inception. The first few cases occurred around mid-December, most likely some time between December 12 and December 30. They began in Wuhan, China, located in the Hubei province, and slowly spread outwards. At the time, they were believed to be average upper respiratory infections of unknown origin, occasionally leading to cases of pneumonia. Initially they seemed like very little to be concerned about, until more people began to become ill. When the virus began to spread faster and further than anticipated, it became an illness that was of great concern. The unknown sickness was reported to the WHO on December 31.

Though December is the month of the virus' origin, very little is known about its progress from official sources during this time. This is because it was not reported until the very end of December, which gave the virus at least a few weeks to fester and spread before most people knew of its existence. Some people have raised concerns with this estimation, claiming that Chinese governments had known about the virus earlier than what they reported, or that even if the stated time frame is correct that the government should have worked faster to quarantine and report the new virus. While we cannot be sure how early the possibility of an outbreak was known, we can get a good sense of the importance of rapid reporting. Had those in charge reacted immediately, perhaps we would not have seen quite the extent of spread that we are currently experiencing. However, since the virus masqueraded as a standard upper respiratory tract infection and only developed to pneumonia symptoms in a few people and after a few days had passed, it may have been hard to mount a response any faster than what already occurred. After all, it is hard to recognize a potential outbreak situation until you are standing in the middle of it, and most doctors diagnosing illnesses likely would not have assumed the cases were anything different from what they had experienced before.

There is no way to go back in time and recognize the mid-December cases for the serious new virus they heralded. As such, we may never be certain if a faster response was possible, or if it would have turned the coronavirus into something that was only a short blip in the news, forgotten as quickly as it arrived. Still, we can use our current circumstances to yield better results the next time a similar situation occurs. Outbreaks and epidemics will continue to appear, and with each new occurrence, we can choose how we react to the potential threat. The possible delay in taking the coronavirus seriously means that it has spread quickly this time, but should we be in the same situation again, the experience may encourage those who must report new cases of unknown origin to act faster so that next time more lives can be saved.

January 2020

January was the first time most people outside of China began to hear about this new virus. At first, it all seemed very far away, and a minor cause for concern if any. However, as the month progressed, people began to grow more and more concerned about the virus crossing country borders and spreading to different nations. The coronavirus started to gain traction in the news and people outside of China started to wonder if this illness might infect them or their loved ones. Still, the level of concern was generally relatively low, as we still did not know much about the virus. Its speed of spread, mortality rate, and likelihood of becoming a serious issue was still unknown. If there was one overarching theme of January, it was uncertainty. We simply did not have all the information yet.

Despite there being just as many people downplaying concerns as there were people suggesting we were about to experience an apocalypse, the coronavirus was starting to become a legitimate concern for many people. In January, the virus affected people in various countries including Japan, Thailand, and the United States. The majority of these cases were a result of travel to an affected area, with the traveler falling ill and potentially passing the virus on to others they had come in contact with since returning home. Since it was beginning to look like the virus would impact many areas of the world, the coronavirus was considered a global problem by the end of the month, though many who lived in unaffected areas still had their doubts about just how likely it was for them to be infected.

The following section breaks down the month into shorter periods and examines each to get a good idea of how the virus developed throughout the first month of 2020.

Early January

At the beginning of the month, people were hard at work identifying a possible source of the new illness. Many cases had been traced back to a market in Wuhan, which was shortly closed to prevent further transmission from the original source. Little is known about the cases of pneumonia, except that they were not caused by the same virus that was responsible for previous SARS or MERS outbreaks. On January 7, Chinese authorities named the illness the product of a coronavirus, suggesting a potential new strain that had not been seen before. The strain was isolated and sequencing efforts began so that the genetic code could be shared with researchers around the globe. The novel coronavirus was dubbed 2019-nCoV, its first official name given by the WHO. Reported cases continued to escalate in number and severity, with many more developing into pneumonia as time went on and an immediate treatment was not found. Still, the coronavirus remained non-fatal for a few more days.

This changed on January 11th, when the first death was announced. According to the Wuhan Municipal Health Commission, "A 61-year-old man, exposed to the virus at the seafood market, died on January 9 after respiratory failure caused by severe pneumonia" (CNN Editorial

Research, 2020, para. 7). Though the death was reported to have occurred on the 9th, it was not reported until two days later. It is unclear if this delay was a purposeful attempt to minimize panic surrounding the virus or if it was simply the product of too much information being exchanged and the report from a single hospital not making it through to official notice until a few days had passed.

Now that it had been proven that the coronavirus was capable of escalating to something deadly, even if only in rare cases, many people were beginning to see the virus as a legitimate threat. It was unclear what factors, if any, might have made someone more susceptible to dying from the infection. Because of this, a great deal of worry and fear spread through those who had heard of the new deadly virus coming out of China, and media coverage of 2019-nCoV started to escalate.

Mid-January

As January progressed, the virus started to cause infections in countries other than China. The first country to be hit was Thailand, which reported its first case on January 13. The person in question had recently traveled to Wuhan, suggesting direct contact with the virus had occurred. Reports followed on January 16, 20, and 21 of cases in Japan, the Republic of Korea, and the United States respectively. The US case occurred in California. Two more deaths occurred in China at this time, the first on January 17 and the second on January 20. The virus' footholds in other countries continued to be minimal, though still at a high risk of spreading to many more people. By January 20, 314 cases of coronavirus had been reported worldwide (WHO, 2020-a, para. 1). While the virus was starting to become more concerning, all cases in other countries were a result of travel from China, so the virus had not yet started to spread between people in other countries.

Despite an increased spread of the virus, mid-January also brought about a great deal of research. On January 12, the novel coronavirus' genetic code was fully sequenced and quickly released for other countries to use for diagnosing potential cases. This likely led to the ability to confirm cases in other countries, which may be why this was around the same time when Thailand, Japan, the Republic of Korea, and the US started to report their first cases. While the growing spread was concerning, these advancements in doctors' abilities to diagnose the coronavirus accurately likely helped to save many lives by containing people who were known to have the virus and getting them the treatment they needed.

Late January

Late January brought with it the beginning of travel restrictions and quarantines in an attempt to control the reach of the coronavirus. China began closing airport and railway stations out of Wuhan, initially on a temporary basis, to try to keep the spread contained. Many Lunar New Year celebrations were canceled, notably those to be held in Beijing, and cities surrounding Wuhan started to restrict travel and transport as well. Vietnam and the Republic of Singapore had joined the list of countries with confirmed cases by January 24; Australia followed shortly after, joined by many more nations from the Philippines to Italy. Other countries with at least one case of coronavirus by the end of January included Germany, Malaysia, France, India, and the United Arab Emirates.

As the situation worsened in China and worry grew in other nations, the US decided to start refusing entry to non-US residents who had traveled to China in the last two weeks. Theoretically, this would prevent further US cases of coronavirus, but by January 30 a case of person-to-person transfer of the virus within the US was reported, meaning there could already be many more people incubating the virus in their systems. This is the same day that the WHO declared the virus a PHEIC, making it a global issue, just seven days after it had ruled against the designation.

The virus took very little time to start making foreign governments very concerned very quickly.

Despite this period seeing the beginnings of quarantines and restrictions on travel between countries, it also saw increased aid from foreign nations looking to stop or slow the outbreak in China. Experts from across the globe lent aid to China and the city of Wuhan specifically in an international task force hoping to examine the issues and provide help where they could. The US also created its own task force for keeping track of the virus and monitoring those who had fallen ill. Official organizations continued to reassure that halting the spread of the virus was possible "provided that countries put in place strong measures to detect disease early, isolate and treat cases, trace contacts, and promote social distancing measures commensurate with the risk" (WHO, 2020-b, para. 1). Still, things were not looking ideal for those fighting against the virus, as the number of global cases was now over 9800. Many of the cases had been spread throughout local communities with no direct contact with Wuhan.

February 2020

While the coronavirus was well known in China and many other Western Pacific nations in January, it did not really hit many news outlets outside the region until February. As the virus continued to infect people far from its origin point, coverage grew, leading some to grow panicked over the possibility of what they viewed as the next black plague. During February, the virus strengthened its presence in countries outside of China, increasing the number of countries experiencing outbreak situations.

Early February

In early February, the first death outside China occurred. All previous coronavirus related deaths had been inside the country of origin, but this death occurred in the Philippines. Shortly after, the first reports of the virus outside of any country occurred when passengers on the Diamond Princess tested positive for the virus. The cruise ship was instructed to remain at sea to prevent the virus from spreading from the passengers and to ensure every passenger could be tested. Unfortunately, this likely led to many more of the passengers contracting the virus. People were not able to leave the ship until much later in the month.

The Diamond Princess situation made many more concerned about travel and large gatherings during the coronavirus. Big concerts, conventions, and international trips began getting canceled in the interest of restricting virus transmission. Coronavirus concerns interfered with a number of other travel and vacation plans, including many other cruise ships that faced either heavy delays or cancelations.

Towards the end of this period on February 11, the official name of the current coronavirus outbreak changed. Once called 2019-CoV, the virus was now known internationally as COVID-19, and all future reports from organizations like the WHO and CDC began using this name to designate the specific strain in question.

Mid-February

On February 14, the first coronavirus related death in Europe occurred after a Chinese tourist passed away in France. The first case in Africa occurred on the same day, in Egypt. Other countries newly affected during this time period include Canada, the United Kingdom, Russia, Iran, and Spain. Over 600 of the passengers on the Diamond Princess are reported to have contracted the coronavirus. Despite this, on February 19, some of the passengers who tested negative for the virus were allowed to leave the ship. Many cautioned that these people could be potential carriers of the virus even though they had tested negative.

At this time, the WHO began instructing countries on quarantine methods and time periods for international travelers to any infected country, not just China. The organization also continued to instruct health care workers how to best handle patients suspected of having the coronavirus. Many sources noticed growing concerns over the virus in all areas of the world and cautioned people not to devolve into panic, though news coverage began to pick up around mid-February. In the US, the coronavirus had become a frequent subject of conversation as more people were affected by it. Many people worried that their state would be the next to report a coronavirus case if it hadn't already. Around this same time, concerns over prejudice and stereotyping fueled by coronavirus panic began to grow.

Late February

By late February, many researchers and scientists had started to work on possible treatments and cures for the virus. These included trial runs of new antiviral medications, using vaccines that target similar illnesses to see if any would have an impact on the coronavirus, and the beginnings of the development of a coronavirus vaccine. However, many have cautioned that a vaccine would not be ready for public distribution for many months, and potentially not until the coronavirus outbreak has already ended.

Concerns over viral transmission between unrelated members of the community, known as community spread, started to occur during this time. People who tested positive for the virus often had no known connection to other infected patients, meaning they likely picked it up through being in a public space with someone with the virus or by touching an infected surface. The growing concerns over community spread led to more frequent and more common quarantines that attempted to keep the affected areas to a minimum.

One notably strict quarantine occurred in Italy as the nation faced an outbreak that was starting to become very severe. Many towns entered into total lockdown as the virus' reach expanded. Both Iran and Japan started to have many more confirmed cases around this time as well. The virus was no longer only a major issue in China. While overall numbers of infection cases were not as high in the US, on February 29, the first US death due to coronavirus occurred.

March 2020

March has been a month of new developments and continued spread. By the beginning of the month, there were over 87,000 confirmed cases of coronavirus globally, with the vast majority of those cases, about 80,000 of them, occurring in China (WHO, 2020-c, para. 5). Around the globe and in the US specifically, public schools and universities are beginning to close, and many businesses have started to suggest that employees work from home to reduce the risk of spreading the virus throughout the company. Multiple US states have declared states of emergency. Many people have flocked to the stores to purchase supplies, both helpful and less so, spurred on by growing concern and doomsday-esque coverage that incites panic. The number of countries reporting confirmed coronavirus cases continues to grow, as does the number of people infected in each of these countries.

Despite an increased spread in many areas, conditions in China actually seem to be improving. China has reported that many of their patients have made recoveries and that there is not nearly as much medical treatment needed now as there was a few months ago. Many of the temporary hospitals constructed during the height of the outbreak have started to close, suggesting that they are no longer necessary. These improvements in China point towards an end to the coronavirus, though we cannot yet be sure exactly when that end will come or what kind of spread to expect in other countries before it happens.

It is uncertain what the future holds and how much worse the coronavirus situation will get before it gets better. As March continues, there will likely be many more new cases, especially in the US where the virus' presence is still relatively low but starting to appear on both coasts and in states across the country. However, this does not mean we should start expecting the worst and giving up on the virus ever going away. March has also brought with it an outpouring of support for those affected, an improvement in public knowledge about the virus, and strong solidarity with medical professionals of all nations as they cooperate to keep the coronavirus from affecting as many lives as possible.

Though times look tough, we do not have to assume the future is grim; banding together, sharing accurate information from verified sources rather than encouraging fear mongering, and practicing good habits for staying safe and healthy are all ways we can each do our part to limit the spread of the virus and better prepare for future outbreaks.

Conclusion

Outbreaks and epidemics are strenuous situations. It can be hard to face the idea that there is an illness that currently has no known cure, and even harder to think that it might be affecting people in your area if it has no already. Concern for yourself, your family, and your community members is natural and expected. This is especially true for countries that have not been as heavily affected by previous coronavirus outbreaks like SARS and MERS, as there is less public knowledge about these viruses and less experience dealing with them. A lack of accurate, verified information can make panic even worse, especially when so much misinformation is involved in a great deal of the coronavirus coverage. Though all of this can make it tempting to give in to your concern and start predicting the apocalypse is upon us, resist the urge to fall victim to fatalistic thinking.

Facing the coronavirus with a level headed understanding of what has happened so far and what is likely to happen next is the best way to ensure you are taking the right steps. Don't rush to the stores to buy up all the overpriced boxes of face masks that will do little to actually keep you healthy; follow health guidelines and focus on washing your hands after being in a public space and limiting the number of times you touch your face. Don't be tricked by false advertisements of products claiming to cure you or make you immune; recognize these for the fraudulent products they are and wait until an official vaccine or antiviral medication has been released. Above all else, don't be fooled into believing that the coronavirus outbreak will last forever. Like all other outbreaks that the human race has experienced, cases will begin to dwindle, people will start to recover, and life will return to normal. The beginnings of the end are already visible in China, and though we cannot be sure just how much longer the virus will be around in other countries, seeing it loosen its grip on the most heavily impacted nation certainly provides a reason to be hopeful for the future.

Facing the Future

The coronavirus is not the first outbreak mankind has faced, and it almost certainly will not be the last. There is always a risk of a future threat, whether viral in nature or from another source entirely. It is not always easy to weather these storms, or to accept that more may be coming in the future. They can bring with them great fear for those waiting for the next great disaster to occur, and great suffering and loss for those who are affected. Though these times can be hard, it is not time to give up. If we all simply stopped fighting the coronavirus, stopped trying to keep ourselves virus-free and refrained from doing any tests or quarantines to keep the virus at bay, we would have thousands more cases than we do now. While healthy people may be able to fend off the virus, they would likely infect many more immunocompromised people who would be unable to do the same. It is only through a joint effort with cooperation from everyone and care for our fellow community members that we can be sure we will defeat this stumbling block and whatever problems come next.

We cannot know what the future holds, but we can be as prepared as possible for the next viral sickness or other hardship. We can learn from the coronavirus and epidemics of the past, as many researchers have done this year, and use them to inform our decisions, keeping what works and discouraging what doesn't. Whatever new threats may await us, knowledge and calm, rational thought will help us overcome it. Pessimistic thinking and giving up is simply not an option. When we support people affected by a tragedy and come together from all nations to stop the spread of diseases, we minimize the impact of harmful myths, clear up any misconceptions that may stand in the way of proper treatment, and give everyone the information and support they need to succeed in the face of any threat.

References

Amar, N. (2020, Feb. 11). "We sing this song for you, Wuhan!": A short history of

Wuhan punk. Retrieved March 10, 2020, from https://radiichina.com/

wuhan-punk-history/

Branswell, H. (2020, Jan. 30). Limited data may be skewing assumptions about severity

of coronavirus outbreak, experts say. Retrieved March 7, 2020, from

https://www.statnews.com/2020/ 01/30/limited-data-may-skew-assumptions-

severity-coronavirus-outbreak/

CDC. (2019, Aug. 2). Middle East Respiratory Syndrome (MERS). Retrieved March 4,

2020, from https://www.cdc.gov/coronavirus/mers/about/index.html

CNN Editorial Research. (2020, Mar. 11). Coronavirus outbreak timeline fast facts.

Retrieved March 11, 2020, from https://www.cnn.com/2020/02/06/health/

wuhan-coronavirus-timeline-fast-facts/index.html

Government of Hubei. (2014, Aug. 7). The legend of Yu Boya and Zhong Ziqi. Retrieved

March 9, 2020, from http://en.hubei.gov.cn/culture/intangible/201408/

t20140807_512476.shtml

Harmsen, P. (2015, Sep. 16). The US Firebombing of Wuhan, Part 2. Retrieved from

http://www.chinaww2.com/2015/09/16/the-us-firebombing-of-wuhan-part-2/

Harrison, S. (2020, Mar. 3). Ask the know-it-alls: What is the coronavirus? Retrieved March 5, 2020, from https://www.wired.com/story/what-is-a-coronavirus/

Hollingsworth, J., (2020, Mar. 5). There's no evidence your pet can get sick from coronavirus. Here's why one dog tested positive. Retrieved March 8, 2020, from https://www.cnn.com/2020/03/02/asia/pets-coronavirus-spread-intl-hnk/index.html

Keyser, Zachary. (2020, Mar. 3). Iranian MPs, health officials claim Tehran is under-reporting coronavirus. Retrieved March 7, 2020, from https://www.jpost.com/Middle-East/Iranian-MPs-health-officials-claim-Tehran-is-underreporting-coronavirus-619604

Levitt, A. (2020, Feb. 7). When you think of Wuhan, think of hot dry noodles. Retrieved

March 10, 2020, from https://thetakeout.com/wuhan-hot-dry-noodles-

coronavirus-1841519191

NIH. (2020, Mar. 6). In the news: Coronavirus and "alternative" treatments. Retrieved

March 7, 2020, from https://nccih.nih.gov/health/in-the-news-in-the-news-

coronavirus-and-alternative-treatments

Taylor, A. (2020, Mar. 4). Congressional negotiators reach $8.3 billion bipartisan

agreement to battle coronavirus. Retrieved March 5, 2020, from

https://time.com/5795748/congress-coronavirus-bill/

WHO. (2020-a, Jan. 20). Novel coronavirus (2019-nCoV) situation report - 1. Retrieved

March 11, 2020, from https://www.who.int/docs/default-source/coronaviruse/

situation-reports/20200121-sitrep-1-2019-ncov.pdf?sfvrsn=20a99c10_4

WHO. (2020-b, Jan. 31). Novel coronavirus (2019-nCoV) situation report - 11. Retrieved

March 11, 2020, from https://www.who.int/docs/default-source/coronaviruse/

situation-reports/20200131-sitrep-11-ncov.pdf?sfvrsn=de7c0f7_4

WHO. (2020-c, Feb. 2). Novel coronavirus (2019-nCoV) situation report - 13. Retrieved

March 11, 2020, from https://www.who.int/docs/default-source/coronaviruse/

situation-reports/20200202-
sitrep-13-ncov-v3.pdf?sfvrsn=195f4010_6

WHO. (2020-d, Jan. 3). Statement on the second meeting of the International Health

Regulations (2005) Emergency Committee regarding the outbreak of novel

coronavirus (2019-nCoV). Retrieved March 6, 2020, from

https://www.who.int/news-room/detail/30-01-2020-statement-on-the-second-

meeting-of-the-international-health-regulations-(2005)-emergency-committee-

regarding-the-outbreak-of-novel-coronavirus-(2019-ncov)

Yu, X. (2020, Feb. 5). My hometown is being ravaged by the coronavirus. Retrieved

March 10, 2020, from https://www.theatlantic.com/ideas/archive/2020/02/

watching-coronavirus-take-over-wuhan-my-hometown/606106/